LIVER CLEANSE DIET RECIPES FOR WOMEN

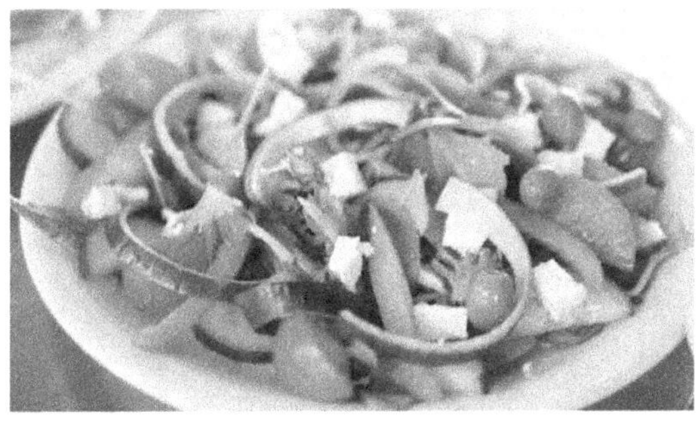

DR. JESSICA SMITH

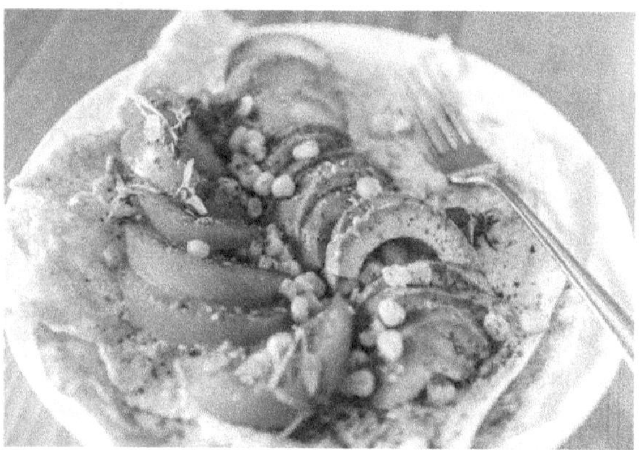

TABLE OF CONTENTS

CHAPTER ONE

How to Use this Cookbook

Understand the Basics: Learn about the liver cleanse diet and its benefits for women. Research reliable sources or consult a healthcare professional to understand how it works and what foods are beneficial.

Consult a Healthcare Professional: Before starting any new diet or cleanse, it's essential to consult with your healthcare provider, especially if you have any existing medical conditions or concerns.

Choose Fresh, Whole Foods: Opt for fresh fruits, vegetables, whole grains, lean proteins, and healthy fats. Avoid processed foods, sugary snacks, and excessive amounts of caffeine and alcohol.

Hydrate: Drink plenty of water throughout the day to help flush out toxins from your system and support liver function. You can also include herbal teas and infused water for variety.

Incorporate Liver-Friendly Foods: Include foods that are known to support liver health, such as leafy greens (kale, spinach), cruciferous vegetables (broccoli, Brussels sprouts), garlic, onions, beets, apples, and berries.

Limit Toxins: Reduce your exposure to toxins by choosing organic produce when possible and avoiding processed foods with additives and preservatives. Minimize alcohol intake and quit smoking if applicable.

Try Liver Cleanse Recipes: Experiment with liver cleanse recipes that incorporate liver-friendly ingredients. Examples include green smoothies with spinach, kale, and apple, roasted beets with garlic, and quinoa salad with avocado and lemon dressing.

Include Detoxifying Herbs and Spices: Incorporate herbs and spices known for their detoxifying properties, such as turmeric, ginger, cilantro, and dandelion greens, into your recipes for added flavor and health benefits.

Balance Macronutrients: Ensure your meals contain a balance of carbohydrates, protein, and healthy fats to provide sustained energy and support overall health. Aim for variety and colorful plates.

Monitor How You Feel: Pay attention to how your body responds to the liver cleanse diet.

Note any changes in energy levels, digestion, and overall well-being. Adjust your diet as needed and continue to prioritize whole, nutrient-dense foods for long-term health.

Understanding Liver Cleanse Diet for Women

Understanding the liver cleanse diet for women involves grasping its principles, benefits, and implementation tailored to female health needs.

The liver plays a crucial role in detoxification, metabolism, and hormone regulation, particularly relevant to women's health due to unique hormonal fluctuations and metabolic demands.

The liver cleanse diet aims to support liver function, enhance detoxification processes, and promote overall well-being through dietary adjustments.

Key principles of the liver cleanse diet include consuming nutrient-dense whole foods, minimizing exposure to toxins, and staying hydrated.

Emphasis is placed on incorporating liver-friendly foods rich in antioxidants, vitamins, and minerals, such as leafy greens, cruciferous vegetables, fruits, lean proteins, and healthy fats.

These foods provide essential nutrients that aid in liver detoxification pathways and support hormone balance.

Benefits of the liver cleanse diet for women may include improved digestion, increased energy levels, clearer skin, and better hormonal balance.

By reducing the intake of processed foods, alcohol, and caffeine while prioritizing whole, plant-based foods, women can support their liver's ability to metabolize hormones effectively and eliminate toxins from the body.

It's important for women to consult healthcare professionals before starting any new diet, including a liver cleanse, especially if they have underlying health conditions or are pregnant or breastfeeding.

Listening to one's body and making gradual dietary changes can lead to sustainable improvements in liver health and overall wellness.

Benefits of Liver Cleanse Diet for Women

The liver cleanse diet offers several benefits specifically tailored to women's health, addressing unique physiological needs and promoting overall well-being. Here are some key advantages:

Hormonal Balance: Women undergo various hormonal fluctuations throughout their lives, from menstrual cycles to pregnancy and menopause.

A liver cleanse diet can help support hormone balance by aiding in the metabolism and elimination of excess hormones, reducing symptoms of hormonal imbalances such as PMS and menopausal symptoms.

Improved Digestion: The liver plays a vital role in digestion by producing bile, which helps break down fats. A diet focused on liver health can improve digestion, reduce bloating, and alleviate digestive discomfort, leading to better nutrient absorption and overall gut health.

Enhanced Detoxification: The liver is the body's primary detoxification organ, responsible for filtering toxins from the bloodstream. By consuming a diet rich in antioxidants, vitamins, and minerals, women can support the liver's detoxification processes, leading to improved toxin elimination and reduced oxidative stress.

Increased Energy Levels: A healthy liver is essential for energy metabolism, as it stores and releases glucose as needed. By optimizing liver function through a cleanse diet, women may experience increased energy levels, reduced fatigue, and improved vitality.

Clearer Skin: The liver cleanse diet can promote clearer, healthier skin by reducing the body's toxic burden and supporting liver function. By eliminating processed foods and consuming nutrient-dense whole foods, women may notice improvements in skin complexion, texture, and overall appearance.

The liver cleanse diet offers women a natural and holistic approach to supporting liver health, hormone balance, digestion, and overall vitality.

However, it's essential to approach any dietary changes with caution and consult healthcare professionals for personalized guidance and advice.

Guidelines for Liver Cleanse Diet for Women

Following guidelines for a liver cleanse diet tailored to women can optimize its effectiveness and ensure overall health benefits.

Here are some key guidelines to consider:

Consultation with Healthcare Professional: Before embarking on any dietary cleanse, especially one targeting the liver, women should consult with a healthcare professional.

This step is crucial for assessing individual health status, identifying any potential contraindications, and obtaining personalized advice.

Focus on Whole Foods: Base the diet on whole, nutrient-dense foods such as fruits, vegetables, whole grains, lean proteins, and healthy fats. These foods provide essential nutrients and antioxidants that support liver function and overall health.

Hydration: Stay well-hydrated by drinking plenty of water throughout the day. Hydration supports detoxification processes and helps flush toxins from the body.

Limit Processed Foods and Toxins: Minimize intake of processed foods, refined sugars, artificial additives, alcohol, and caffeine. These substances can burden the liver and hinder its ability to detoxify effectively.

Liver-Friendly Foods: Incorporate foods known to support liver health, such as leafy greens, cruciferous vegetables, garlic, onions, beets, apples, berries, and herbs like turmeric and ginger.

Moderate Protein Intake: Include moderate amounts of lean protein sources, such as poultry, fish, tofu, beans, and legumes, to support liver function and muscle maintenance.

Reduce Environmental Toxins: Take steps to minimize exposure to environmental toxins by choosing organic produce, using natural cleaning and personal care products, and avoiding exposure to pollutants and chemicals whenever possible.

Monitor Portion Sizes: Pay attention to portion sizes and avoid overeating. Eating smaller, balanced meals throughout the day can help maintain stable blood sugar levels and support digestion.

Practice Mindful Eating: Eat slowly, chew food thoroughly, and pay attention to hunger and fullness cues. Mindful eating can promote better digestion and prevent overeating.

CHAPTER TWO

Liver Cleanse Breakfast Diet Recipes for Women

1: Green Detox Smoothie

Ingredients:

- 1 cup spinach
- 1/2 cup kale, stems removed
- 1/2 cucumber, peeled and chopped
- 1/2 green apple, cored and chopped
- 1/2 lemon, juiced
- 1 tablespoon fresh ginger, grated
- 1 cup coconut water or filtered water
- Optional: 1 tablespoon chia seeds or flaxseeds for added fiber and omega-3 fatty acids

Instructions:

- Add all ingredients to a blender.
- Blend until smooth and creamy.
- If the smoothie is too thick, add more water to reach your desired consistency.

- Pour into a glass and enjoy immediately.

Health Benefits:

- Spinach and kale are rich in chlorophyll, which can help support liver detoxification.
- Cucumber and lemon provide hydration and are alkalizing to the body.
- Ginger has anti-inflammatory properties and aids digestion.
- Apples add natural sweetness and are a good source of fiber and antioxidants.
- Chia seeds or flaxseeds add omega-3 fatty acids and additional fiber for digestive health.

Preparation Time: 5 minutes

2: Quinoa Breakfast Bowl

Ingredients:

- 1/2 cup cooked quinoa
- 1/4 cup mixed berries (such as strawberries, blueberries, raspberries)
- 1 tablespoon pumpkin seeds
- 1 tablespoon unsweetened coconut flakes

- 1 tablespoon hemp seeds

- 1/4 teaspoon cinnamon

- 1/2 cup unsweetened almond milk or coconut milk

Instructions:

- In a bowl, layer cooked quinoa.

- Top with mixed berries, pumpkin seeds, coconut flakes, and hemp seeds.

- Sprinkle cinnamon over the bowl.

- Pour almond milk or coconut milk over the ingredients.

- Stir gently to combine.

- Enjoy your nutritious breakfast bowl!

Health Benefits:

- Quinoa is a complete protein and contains fiber, vitamins, and minerals.

- Berries are rich in antioxidants, which support liver health and overall well-being.

- Pumpkin seeds and hemp seeds provide protein, healthy fats, and essential nutrients.

- Cinnamon helps regulate blood sugar levels and adds a warm, comforting flavor.
- Coconut flakes add healthy fats and a touch of sweetness.

Preparation Time: 10 minutes

3: Avocado Toast with Turmeric

Ingredients:

- 1 ripe avocado
- 2 slices whole grain bread or gluten-free bread
- 1/2 teaspoon ground turmeric
- 1/2 teaspoon black pepper (to enhance turmeric absorption)
- Pinch of sea salt
- Optional toppings: sliced tomato, microgreens, radish slices, or poached egg

Instructions:

- Toast the bread slices until golden brown.
- While the bread is toasting, mash the ripe avocado in a bowl.

- Mix in the ground turmeric, black pepper, and a pinch of sea salt.
- Once the bread is toasted, spread the mashed avocado mixture evenly on each slice.
- Add optional toppings such as sliced tomato, microgreens, radish slices, or a poached egg.
- Sprinkle with additional black pepper if desired.
- Serve immediately and enjoy!

Health Benefits:

- Avocado is rich in healthy fats and fiber, which support liver health and digestion.
- Turmeric contains curcumin, a compound with powerful anti-inflammatory and antioxidant properties that may help support liver function.
- Black pepper enhances the absorption of curcumin in turmeric.
- Whole grain bread provides complex carbohydrates and fiber for sustained energy.

Preparation Time: 10 minutes

4: Berry Chia Seed Pudding

Ingredients:

- 1/4 cup chia seeds
- 1 cup unsweetened almond milk or coconut milk
- 1/2 teaspoon pure vanilla extract
- 1 tablespoon maple syrup or honey (optional, for sweetness)
- 1/2 cup mixed berries (such as strawberries, blueberries, raspberries)
- 1 tablespoon unsweetened coconut flakes

Instructions:

- In a bowl or jar, mix together chia seeds, almond milk (or coconut milk), vanilla extract, and maple syrup (if using).
- Stir well to combine, ensuring there are no clumps of chia seeds.
- Cover and refrigerate for at least 2 hours or overnight, allowing the chia seeds to absorb the liquid and thicken.
- Once the chia pudding has set, remove it from the refrigerator.

- Top with mixed berries and unsweetened coconut flakes.
- Serve chilled and enjoy!

Health Benefits:

- Chia seeds are rich in omega-3 fatty acids, fiber, and protein, which support heart health, digestion, and satiety.
- Berries provide antioxidants, vitamins, and minerals that support liver detoxification and overall health.
- Unsweetened almond milk or coconut milk adds creaminess without added sugars.
- Vanilla extract adds flavor without additional calories or sugars.

Preparation Time: 5 minutes (plus chilling time)

5: Turmeric Ginger Smoothie Bowl

Ingredients:

- 1 frozen banana
- 1/2 cup frozen pineapple chunks
- 1/2 cup spinach
- 1 teaspoon grated fresh ginger

- 1/2 teaspoon ground turmeric
- 1/2 cup unsweetened almond milk or coconut milk
- Toppings: sliced kiwi, coconut flakes, chia seeds, granola

Instructions:

- In a blender, combine the frozen banana, frozen pineapple chunks, spinach, grated ginger, ground turmeric, and almond milk.
- Blend until smooth and creamy, adding more almond milk if needed to reach your desired consistency.
- Pour the smoothie into a bowl.
- Top with sliced kiwi, coconut flakes, chia seeds, and granola.
- Serve immediately and enjoy with a spoon!

Health Benefits:

- Turmeric and ginger both have anti-inflammatory properties that support liver health and reduce inflammation in the body.
- Spinach adds fiber, vitamins, and minerals to support overall health and digestion.

- Kiwi provides vitamin C and antioxidants, which support immune function and detoxification.
- Chia seeds and granola add texture, fiber, and healthy fats for sustained energy.

Preparation Time: 5 minutes

6: Veggie Omelette with Herbs

Ingredients:

- 2 eggs
- 1/4 cup diced bell peppers (any color)
- 1/4 cup diced tomatoes
- 1/4 cup diced mushrooms
- 1 tablespoon chopped fresh herbs (such as parsley, basil, or cilantro)
- 1 teaspoon olive oil or coconut oil
- Salt and pepper to taste

Instructions:

- In a bowl, beat the eggs until well combined. Season with salt and pepper.
- Heat olive oil or coconut oil in a non-stick skillet over medium heat.

- Add diced bell peppers, tomatoes, and mushrooms to the skillet. Sauté until softened, about 3-4 minutes.
- Pour the beaten eggs over the sautéed vegetables in the skillet.
- Cook the omelette until the edges are set and the center is slightly runny, about 2-3 minutes.
- Sprinkle chopped fresh herbs over one half of the omelette.
- Using a spatula, fold the other half of the omelette over the herb-covered half.
- Cook for another 1-2 minutes until the eggs are fully cooked through.
- Slide the omelette onto a plate and serve hot.

Health Benefits:

- Eggs are a good source of protein, vitamins, and minerals, including choline, which supports liver health and metabolism.
- Bell peppers, tomatoes, and mushrooms provide vitamins, minerals, and antioxidants that support overall health and detoxification.

- Fresh herbs add flavor and provide additional nutrients and antioxidants.

Preparation Time: 10 minutes

7: Overnight Oats with Berries and Almonds

Ingredients:

- 1/2 cup rolled oats
- 1/2 cup unsweetened almond milk or coconut milk
- 1/4 cup Greek yogurt (or dairy-free alternative)
- 1 tablespoon chia seeds
- 1/4 teaspoon pure vanilla extract
- 1/2 cup mixed berries (such as strawberries, blueberries, raspberries)
- 1 tablespoon sliced almonds
- Optional: drizzle of honey or maple syrup for sweetness

Instructions:

- In a jar or bowl, combine rolled oats, almond milk (or coconut milk), Greek yogurt, chia seeds, and vanilla extract.
- Stir well to combine all ingredients.

- Gently fold in mixed berries and sliced almonds.
- Cover the jar or bowl and refrigerate overnight, or for at least 4 hours, to allow the oats to soften and the flavors to meld.
- Before serving, give the oats a stir and add a drizzle of honey or maple syrup if desired.
- Enjoy your creamy and nutritious overnight oats!

Health Benefits:

- Oats are rich in fiber, which supports digestion and helps remove toxins from the body.
- Almond milk or coconut milk provides healthy fats and is dairy-free, making it suitable for those with lactose intolerance or dairy allergies.
- Greek yogurt adds protein and probiotics, which support gut health and digestion.
- Berries are packed with antioxidants, vitamins, and minerals that support liver detoxification and overall health.
- Chia seeds add omega-3 fatty acids and additional fiber for sustained energy.

Preparation Time: 5 minutes (plus chilling time)

Ingredients:

- 1 large whole grain or gluten-free tortilla
- 2 eggs, beaten
- 1 cup fresh spinach leaves
- 1/2 cup sliced mushrooms
- 1/4 cup diced tomatoes
- 1/4 cup shredded mozzarella cheese or dairy-free alternative
- 1 teaspoon olive oil or coconut oil
- Salt and pepper to taste
- Optional: salsa or avocado slices for serving

Instructions:

- Heat olive oil or coconut oil in a skillet over medium heat.
- Add sliced mushrooms to the skillet and sauté until softened, about 3-4 minutes.
- Add beaten eggs to the skillet and scramble until cooked through.
- Season the eggs with salt and pepper to taste.

- Lay the tortilla flat on a plate or cutting board.

- Place fresh spinach leaves on the tortilla, followed by scrambled eggs, diced tomatoes, and shredded mozzarella cheese.

- Roll up the tortilla tightly to form a wrap.

- If desired, heat the wrap in the skillet for 1-2 minutes on each side until lightly toasted.

- Slice the wrap in half and serve with salsa or avocado slices on the side.

Health Benefits:

- Spinach is rich in chlorophyll, which supports liver detoxification and overall health.

- Mushrooms provide antioxidants and B vitamins that support immune function and energy metabolism.

- Eggs are a good source of protein, vitamins, and minerals, including choline, which supports liver health and metabolism.

- Whole grain tortillas add fiber and complex carbohydrates for sustained energy.

- Tomatoes add vitamins, minerals, and antioxidants, such as lycopene, which supports heart health and detoxification.

Preparation Time: 15 minutes

9: Beet and Berry Smoothie

Ingredients:

- 1 small beet, peeled and chopped
- 1/2 cup mixed berries (such as strawberries, blueberries, raspberries)
- 1/2 banana
- 1/2 cup plain Greek yogurt or dairy-free alternative
- 1 tablespoon honey or maple syrup (optional, for sweetness)
- 1/2 cup unsweetened almond milk or coconut milk
- 1 tablespoon chia seeds or ground flaxseeds (optional, for added fiber and omega-3 fatty acids)

Instructions:

- Place the chopped beet, mixed berries, banana, Greek yogurt, honey or maple syrup (if using), and almond milk in a blender.

- Blend until smooth and creamy.

- If the smoothie is too thick, add more almond milk to reach your desired consistency.

- Add chia seeds or ground flaxseeds if desired and blend briefly to incorporate.

- Pour the smoothie into a glass and enjoy immediately.

Health Benefits:

- Beets contain betalains, which support liver detoxification and have anti-inflammatory properties.

- Berries are rich in antioxidants, vitamins, and fiber, which support overall health and digestion.

- Banana adds natural sweetness and provides potassium, which supports heart health and electrolyte balance.

- Greek yogurt adds protein and probiotics, which support gut health and digestion.

- Chia seeds or ground flaxseeds add omega-3 fatty acids and additional fiber for digestive health.

Preparation Time: 5 minutes

Ingredients:

- 1 medium sweet potato, peeled and diced
- 1/2 onion, diced
- 1 bell pepper, diced
- 1 cup baby spinach leaves
- 2 eggs
- 1 tablespoon olive oil or coconut oil
- Salt and pepper to taste
- Optional: chopped fresh herbs (such as parsley or cilantro) for garnish

Instructions:

- Heat olive oil or coconut oil in a skillet over medium heat.
- Add diced sweet potato to the skillet and cook until softened and lightly browned, about 5-7 minutes.
- Add diced onion and bell pepper to the skillet and cook until softened, about 3-4 minutes.
- Add baby spinach leaves to the skillet and cook until wilted, about 1-2 minutes.

- Create two wells in the hash mixture and crack an egg into each well.
- Season the eggs with salt and pepper to taste.
- Cover the skillet and cook until the eggs are cooked to your desired doneness, about 3-5 minutes for runny yolks or longer for fully cooked yolks.
- Remove the skillet from heat and sprinkle chopped fresh herbs over the hash.
- Serve hot and enjoy your flavorful sweet potato breakfast hash!

Health Benefits:

- Sweet potatoes are rich in vitamins, minerals, and fiber, which support digestion and liver health.
- Onions and bell peppers provide antioxidants and vitamins that support immune function and overall health.
- Spinach adds chlorophyll, which supports liver detoxification and overall health.
- Eggs are a good source of protein, vitamins, and minerals, including choline, which supports liver health and metabolism.

Preparation Time: 20 minutes

Liver Cleanse Lunch Diet Recipes for Women

1: Quinoa and Roasted Vegetable Salad

Ingredients:

- 1 cup quinoa, rinsed
- 2 cups water or vegetable broth
- 1 small sweet potato, peeled and diced
- 1 small zucchini, sliced
- 1 red bell pepper, diced
- 1 cup cherry tomatoes, halved
- 2 cups mixed greens (spinach, kale, arugula)
- 1/4 cup chopped fresh herbs (such as parsley or cilantro)
- 2 tablespoons olive oil
- 1 tablespoon balsamic vinegar
- Salt and pepper to taste
- Optional: crumbled feta cheese or avocado slices for serving

Instructions:

- Preheat the oven to 400°F (200°C).

- In a saucepan, combine quinoa and water or vegetable broth. Bring to a boil, then reduce heat to low, cover, and simmer for 15-20 minutes until quinoa is tender and water is absorbed.
- While the quinoa is cooking, spread diced sweet potato, sliced zucchini, and diced red bell pepper on a baking sheet. Drizzle with olive oil and sprinkle with salt and pepper. Toss to coat evenly.
- Roast the vegetables in the preheated oven for 20-25 minutes until tender and lightly browned.
- In a large bowl, combine cooked quinoa, roasted vegetables, cherry tomatoes, mixed greens, and chopped fresh herbs.
- Drizzle with balsamic vinegar and toss to coat evenly.
- Divide the salad into serving bowls.
- If desired, top with crumbled feta cheese or avocado slices.
- Serve warm or chilled and enjoy your nourishing quinoa and roasted vegetable salad!

Health Benefits:

- Quinoa is a complete protein and provides fiber, vitamins, and minerals that support digestion and overall health.
- Sweet potatoes, zucchini, bell peppers, and tomatoes are rich in antioxidants, vitamins, and fiber, which support liver detoxification and immune function.
- Mixed greens provide chlorophyll and nutrients that support liver health and digestion.
- Olive oil provides healthy fats and antioxidants, which support heart health and inflammation.
- Balsamic vinegar adds flavor without added sugars or calories.

Preparation Time: 30-35 minutes

2: Lentil and Vegetable Soup

Ingredients:

- 1 cup dried green or brown lentils, rinsed
- 4 cups vegetable broth
- 1 onion, diced
- 2 carrots, diced

- 2 celery stalks, diced

- 2 cloves garlic, minced

- 1 teaspoon ground cumin

- 1/2 teaspoon ground turmeric

- 1/2 teaspoon paprika

- 1 bay leaf

- Salt and pepper to taste

- 2 tablespoons olive oil

- 2 tablespoons lemon juice

- Optional: chopped fresh parsley or cilantro for garnish

Instructions:

- In a large pot, heat olive oil over medium heat.

- Add diced onion, carrots, and celery to the pot. Sauté for 5-7 minutes until vegetables are softened.

- Add minced garlic, ground cumin, ground turmeric, paprika, and bay leaf to the pot. Cook for 1-2 minutes until fragrant.

- Add dried lentils and vegetable broth to the pot. Bring to a boil, then reduce heat to low, cover, and simmer for 20-25 minutes until lentils are tender.

- Once lentils are cooked, remove the bay leaf from the soup.
- Stir in lemon juice and season with salt and pepper to taste.
- Ladle the soup into serving bowls.
- If desired, garnish with chopped fresh parsley or cilantro.
- Serve hot and enjoy your hearty and nutritious lentil and vegetable soup!

Health Benefits:

- Lentils are rich in fiber, protein, and folate, which support digestion, blood sugar regulation, and liver health.
- Onions, carrots, celery, and garlic provide vitamins, minerals, and antioxidants that support immune function and liver detoxification.
- Spices like cumin, turmeric, and paprika have anti-inflammatory properties that support liver health and overall well-being.
- Olive oil provides healthy fats and antioxidants, which support heart health and inflammation.

- Lemon juice adds vitamin C and acidity, which enhance flavor and aid digestion.

Preparation Time: 30-35 minutes

3: Grilled Salmon with Quinoa and Steamed Broccoli

Ingredients:

- 2 salmon fillets
- 1 cup quinoa, rinsed
- 2 cups water or vegetable broth
- 2 cups broccoli florets
- 2 tablespoons olive oil
- 1 lemon, divided
- Salt and pepper to taste
- Optional: chopped fresh dill or parsley for garnish

Instructions:

- Preheat the grill to medium-high heat.
- Season the salmon fillets with salt, pepper, and a squeeze of lemon juice.
- Grill the salmon fillets for 4-5 minutes per side, or until cooked through and flaky.

- While the salmon is grilling, in a saucepan, combine quinoa and water or vegetable broth. Bring to a boil, then reduce heat to low, cover, and simmer for 15-20 minutes until quinoa is tender and water is absorbed.
- In a separate pot, steam broccoli florets until tender, about 5-7 minutes.
- Once the quinoa is cooked, fluff it with a fork and drizzle with olive oil and a squeeze of lemon juice. Season with salt and pepper to taste.
- Divide the cooked quinoa and steamed broccoli onto plates.
- Place grilled salmon fillets on top of the quinoa and broccoli.
- Garnish with chopped fresh dill or parsley if desired.
- Serve hot and enjoy your nutritious grilled salmon with quinoa and steamed broccoli!

Health Benefits:

- Salmon is rich in omega-3 fatty acids, which support heart health and reduce inflammation. It also provides protein and essential nutrients that support overall health.

- Quinoa is a complete protein and contains fiber, vitamins, and minerals that support digestion and liver health.
- Broccoli is rich in antioxidants, fiber, and vitamins, such as vitamin C and vitamin K, which support immune function and liver detoxification.
- Olive oil provides healthy fats and antioxidants, which support heart health and inflammation.
- Lemon juice adds vitamin C and acidity, which enhance flavor and aid digestion.

Preparation Time: 25-30 minutes

4: Chickpea and Avocado Salad

Ingredients:

- 1 can (15 ounces) chickpeas, drained and rinsed
- 1 avocado, diced
- 1 cup cherry tomatoes, halved
- 1/4 cup diced red onion
- 1/4 cup chopped fresh cilantro
- 2 tablespoons olive oil
- 1 tablespoon lemon juice
- 1/2 teaspoon ground cumin

- Salt and pepper to taste
- Optional: crumbled feta cheese or goat cheese for serving

Instructions:

- In a large bowl, combine chickpeas, diced avocado, cherry tomatoes, diced red onion, and chopped fresh cilantro.
- In a small bowl, whisk together olive oil, lemon juice, ground cumin, salt, and pepper to make the dressing.
- Pour the dressing over the chickpea and avocado mixture.
- Gently toss to coat all ingredients evenly.
- If desired, sprinkle crumbled feta cheese or goat cheese over the salad before serving.
- Serve chilled or at room temperature and enjoy your flavorful chickpea and avocado salad!

Health Benefits:

- Chickpeas are rich in fiber, protein, and vitamins, which support digestion and blood sugar regulation.

They also contain antioxidants and minerals that support liver health.

- Avocado provides healthy fats, fiber, and essential nutrients, such as vitamin E and potassium, which support heart health and inflammation.
- Cherry tomatoes are rich in antioxidants, vitamins, and minerals, such as vitamin C and lycopene, which support immune function and liver detoxification.
- Red onion adds flavor and contains antioxidants and compounds that support heart health and blood sugar regulation.
- Olive oil provides healthy fats and antioxidants, which support heart health and inflammation.

Preparation Time: 15 minutes

5: Quinoa and Black Bean Salad

Ingredients:

- 1 cup quinoa, rinsed
- 2 cups water or vegetable broth
- 1 can (15 ounces) black beans, drained and rinsed
- 1 red bell pepper, diced
- 1 cup corn kernels (fresh or frozen)

- 1/4 cup diced red onion

- 1/4 cup chopped fresh cilantro

- Juice of 2 limes

- 2 tablespoons olive oil

- 1 teaspoon ground cumin

- Salt and pepper to taste

- Optional: diced avocado for serving

Instructions:

- In a saucepan, combine quinoa and water or vegetable broth. Bring to a boil, then reduce heat to low, cover, and simmer for 15-20 minutes until quinoa is tender and water is absorbed.

- In a large bowl, combine cooked quinoa, black beans, diced red bell pepper, corn kernels, diced red onion, and chopped fresh cilantro.

- In a small bowl, whisk together lime juice, olive oil, ground cumin, salt, and pepper to make the dressing.

- Pour the dressing over the quinoa and black bean mixture.

- Gently toss to coat all ingredients evenly.

- If desired, top with diced avocado before serving.

- Serve chilled or at room temperature and enjoy your flavorful quinoa and black bean salad!

Health Benefits:

- Quinoa is a complete protein and contains fiber, vitamins, and minerals that support digestion and liver health.
- Black beans are rich in protein, fiber, and antioxidants, which support heart health and blood sugar regulation. They also contain folate and iron, which support overall health.
- Red bell pepper adds vitamin C and antioxidants, which support immune function and liver detoxification.
- Corn provides fiber and essential nutrients, such as vitamin B6 and potassium, which support digestion and overall health.
- Lime juice adds acidity and flavor while providing vitamin C, which enhances absorption of iron from plant-based foods.

Preparation Time: 25-30 minutes

Ingredients:

- 2 cans (15 ounces each) chickpeas, drained and rinsed
- 1 cucumber, diced
- 1 cup cherry tomatoes, halved
- 1/4 cup diced red onion
- 1/4 cup chopped fresh parsley
- 1/4 cup chopped fresh mint
- Juice of 1 lemon
- 2 tablespoons extra virgin olive oil
- 1 teaspoon dried oregano
- Salt and pepper to taste
- Optional: crumbled feta cheese or olives for serving

Instructions:

- In a large bowl, combine chickpeas, diced cucumber, cherry tomatoes, diced red onion, chopped fresh parsley, and chopped fresh mint.
- In a small bowl, whisk together lemon juice, olive oil, dried oregano, salt, and pepper to make the dressing.

- Pour the dressing over the chickpea salad mixture.

- Gently toss to coat all ingredients evenly.

- If desired, top with crumbled feta cheese or olives before serving.

- Serve chilled or at room temperature and enjoy your refreshing Mediterranean chickpea salad!

Health Benefits:

- Chickpeas are rich in fiber, protein, and vitamins, which support digestion and blood sugar regulation. They also contain antioxidants and minerals that support liver health.

- Cucumber provides hydration and contains antioxidants and compounds that support heart health and inflammation. It also adds freshness and crunch to the salad.

- Cherry tomatoes are rich in antioxidants, vitamins, and minerals, such as vitamin C and lycopene, which support immune function and liver detoxification.

- Red onion adds flavor and contains antioxidants and compounds that support heart health and blood sugar regulation.

- Olive oil provides healthy fats and antioxidants, which support heart health and inflammation.

Preparation Time: 15 minutes

7: Rainbow Veggie Stir-Fry

Ingredients:

- 2 cups mixed vegetables (such as bell peppers, broccoli, carrots, snap peas)
- 1 cup cooked brown rice or quinoa
- 1 tablespoon olive oil
- 2 cloves garlic, minced
- 1 teaspoon grated fresh ginger
- 2 tablespoons low-sodium soy sauce or tamari
- 1 tablespoon rice vinegar
- 1 teaspoon honey or maple syrup (optional)
- Sesame seeds for garnish
- Sliced green onions for garnish

Instructions:

- Heat olive oil in a large skillet or wok over medium-high heat.

- Add minced garlic and grated ginger to the skillet and sauté for 1 minute until fragrant.
- Add mixed vegetables to the skillet and stir-fry for 5-7 minutes until crisp-tender.
- In a small bowl, whisk together soy sauce or tamari, rice vinegar, and honey or maple syrup (if using).
- Pour the sauce over the vegetables in the skillet and toss to coat evenly.
- Add cooked brown rice or quinoa to the skillet and stir-fry for an additional 2-3 minutes until heated through.
- Remove the skillet from heat and garnish with sesame seeds and sliced green onions.
- Serve hot and enjoy your vibrant and nutritious rainbow veggie stir-fry!

Health Benefits:

- Mixed vegetables provide a variety of vitamins, minerals, and antioxidants that support liver health and overall well-being.

- Garlic and ginger have anti-inflammatory and immune-boosting properties that support liver function.

- Brown rice or quinoa provides fiber and complex carbohydrates for sustained energy and digestion.

- Soy sauce or tamari adds savory flavor while providing amino acids and minerals.

- Sesame seeds contain healthy fats and minerals, such as calcium and magnesium, which support bone health and inflammation.

Preparation Time: 20 minutes

8: Tofu and Vegetable Buddha Bowl

Ingredients:

- 1 cup cooked quinoa or brown rice

- 1 cup cubed extra-firm tofu

- 2 cups mixed vegetables (such as broccoli, bell peppers, carrots, cabbage)

- 1 tablespoon olive oil

- 2 tablespoons low-sodium soy sauce or tamari

- 1 tablespoon rice vinegar

- 1 teaspoon grated fresh ginger

- Sesame seeds for garnish
- Sliced green onions for garnish

Instructions:

- Heat olive oil in a large skillet over medium heat.
- Add cubed tofu to the skillet and cook for 5-7 minutes, flipping occasionally, until golden brown and crispy on all sides.
- Remove the tofu from the skillet and set aside.
- In the same skillet, add mixed vegetables and grated fresh ginger. Stir-fry for 5-7 minutes until crisp-tender.
- In a small bowl, whisk together soy sauce or tamari and rice vinegar.
- Return the tofu to the skillet and pour the sauce over the tofu and vegetables. Toss to coat evenly.
- Divide cooked quinoa or brown rice into serving bowls.
- Top with tofu and vegetable mixture from the skillet.
- Garnish with sesame seeds and sliced green onions.
- Serve hot and enjoy your nourishing tofu and vegetable Buddha bowl!

Health Benefits:

- Tofu is a good source of plant-based protein and contains essential amino acids, vitamins, and minerals that support muscle repair and overall health.

- Mixed vegetables provide a variety of vitamins, minerals, and antioxidants that support liver health and overall well-being.

- Quinoa or brown rice adds fiber and complex carbohydrates for sustained energy and digestion.

- Soy sauce or tamari adds savory flavor while providing amino acids and minerals.

- Sesame seeds contain healthy fats and minerals, such as calcium and magnesium, which support bone health and inflammation.

Preparation Time: 25 minutes

9: Mediterranean Chickpea Salad Wrap

Ingredients:

- 1 can (15 ounces) chickpeas, drained and rinsed
- 1 cup cucumber, diced

- 1 cup cherry tomatoes, halved
- 1/4 cup red onion, finely chopped
- 1/4 cup Kalamata olives, pitted and chopped
- 2 tablespoons fresh parsley, chopped
- 2 tablespoons extra virgin olive oil
- 1 tablespoon lemon juice
- 1 teaspoon dried oregano
- Salt and pepper to taste
- 4 whole grain or gluten-free wraps
- Optional: crumbled feta cheese or sliced avocado

Instructions:

- In a large bowl, combine chickpeas, cucumber, cherry tomatoes, red onion, Kalamata olives, and parsley.
- In a small bowl, whisk together olive oil, lemon juice, dried oregano, salt, and pepper to make the dressing.
- Pour the dressing over the chickpea salad and toss until well coated.
- Warm the wraps according to package instructions or preference.

- Divide the chickpea salad evenly among the wraps.
- If desired, top with crumbled feta cheese or sliced avocado.
- Roll up the wraps tightly, slice in half if desired, and serve immediately.

Health Benefits:

- Chickpeas provide protein, fiber, and essential nutrients, supporting digestion and liver health.
- Cucumber and cherry tomatoes are hydrating and provide vitamins, minerals, and antioxidants for overall health.
- Red onion and Kalamata olives add flavor and provide antioxidants and anti-inflammatory compounds.
- Olive oil offers heart-healthy monounsaturated fats and antioxidants that support inflammation and liver health.
- Whole grain wraps provide fiber and complex carbohydrates for sustained energy and digestion.

Preparation Time: 15 minutes

10: Asian-Inspired Tofu Stir-Fry

Ingredients:

- 1 block (14-16 ounces) extra-firm tofu, pressed and cubed
- 2 cups mixed vegetables (such as bell peppers, broccoli, snap peas, carrots)
- 2 cloves garlic, minced
- 1 tablespoon fresh ginger, grated
- 3 tablespoons low-sodium soy sauce or tamari
- 1 tablespoon rice vinegar
- 1 tablespoon honey or maple syrup
- 1 tablespoon sesame oil
- 2 tablespoons vegetable oil (for stir-frying)
- Cooked brown rice or quinoa for serving
- Optional toppings: sliced green onions, sesame seeds, crushed red pepper flakes

Instructions:

- In a small bowl, whisk together soy sauce or tamari, rice vinegar, honey or maple syrup, and sesame oil to make the sauce. Set aside.

- Heat vegetable oil in a large skillet or wok over medium-high heat.
- Add cubed tofu to the skillet and cook until golden brown and crispy on all sides, about 5-7 minutes. Remove tofu from the skillet and set aside.
- In the same skillet, add minced garlic and grated ginger. Stir-fry for 1 minute until fragrant.
- Add mixed vegetables to the skillet and stir-fry for 5-7 minutes until crisp-tender.
- Return the tofu to the skillet and pour the sauce over the tofu and vegetables. Toss until well coated and heated through.
- Serve the tofu stir-fry over cooked brown rice or quinoa.
- Garnish with sliced green onions, sesame seeds, and crushed red pepper flakes if desired.
- Serve hot and enjoy your flavorful Asian-inspired tofu stir-fry!

Health Benefits:

- Tofu provides plant-based protein and essential nutrients, supporting muscle repair and overall health.

- Mixed vegetables offer vitamins, minerals, and antioxidants that support liver health and overall well-being.

- Garlic and ginger contain anti-inflammatory and immune-boosting properties that support liver function.

- Soy sauce or tamari adds savory flavor while providing amino acids and minerals.

- Brown rice or quinoa offers fiber and complex carbohydrates for sustained energy and digestion.

Preparation Time: 25 minutes

Liver Cleanse Dinner Diet Recipes for Women

1: Baked Salmon with Roasted Vegetables

Ingredients:

- 2 salmon fillets

- 2 cups mixed vegetables (such as broccoli, bell peppers, carrots, cauliflower)

- 2 tablespoons olive oil

- 2 cloves garlic, minced

- 1 teaspoon dried thyme

- 1 teaspoon dried rosemary

- Salt and pepper to taste

- Lemon wedges for serving

Instructions:

- Preheat the oven to 400°F (200°C).

- Place salmon fillets on a baking sheet lined with parchment paper.

- In a bowl, toss mixed vegetables with olive oil, minced garlic, dried thyme, dried rosemary, salt, and pepper until evenly coated.

- Spread the vegetables around the salmon fillets on the baking sheet.

- Bake in the preheated oven for 15-20 minutes, or until salmon is cooked through and vegetables are tender.

- Remove from the oven and serve the baked salmon with roasted vegetables.

- Squeeze fresh lemon juice over the salmon before serving.
- Enjoy your nutritious and delicious baked salmon with roasted vegetables!

Health Benefits:

- Salmon is rich in omega-3 fatty acids, which support heart health and reduce inflammation. It also provides protein and essential nutrients that support overall health.
- Mixed vegetables provide a variety of vitamins, minerals, and antioxidants that support liver health and overall well-being.
- Olive oil offers heart-healthy monounsaturated fats and antioxidants that support inflammation and liver health.
- Garlic, thyme, and rosemary contain anti-inflammatory properties and support immune function.

Preparation Time: 25 minutes

2: Quinoa Stuffed Bell Peppers

Ingredients:

- 4 bell peppers, halved and seeds removed
- 1 cup quinoa, rinsed
- 2 cups vegetable broth
- 1 can (15 ounces) black beans, drained and rinsed
- 1 cup corn kernels (fresh or frozen)
- 1 cup cherry tomatoes, halved
- 1/2 cup diced red onion
- 2 cloves garlic, minced
- 1 teaspoon ground cumin
- 1 teaspoon chili powder
- Salt and pepper to taste
- Optional toppings: sliced avocado, chopped fresh cilantro, Greek yogurt or sour cream

Instructions:

- Preheat the oven to 375°F (190°C).
- In a saucepan, combine quinoa and vegetable broth. Bring to a boil, then reduce heat to low, cover, and

simmer for 15-20 minutes until quinoa is tender and liquid is absorbed.

- In a large bowl, combine cooked quinoa, black beans, corn kernels, cherry tomatoes, diced red onion, minced garlic, ground cumin, chili powder, salt, and pepper.
- Fill each halved bell pepper with the quinoa mixture.
- Place stuffed bell peppers in a baking dish.
- Cover the baking dish with foil and bake in the preheated oven for 25-30 minutes, or until bell peppers are tender.
- Remove from the oven and let cool slightly before serving.
- Serve the quinoa stuffed bell peppers with optional toppings such as sliced avocado, chopped fresh cilantro, and Greek yogurt or sour cream.
- Enjoy your flavorful and satisfying quinoa stuffed bell peppers!

Health Benefits:

- Bell peppers are rich in vitamins A and C, antioxidants, and fiber, which support immune function and liver detoxification.
- Quinoa provides protein, fiber, and essential nutrients, supporting digestion and liver health.
- Black beans offer protein, fiber, and antioxidants, supporting heart health and blood sugar regulation.
- Corn provides fiber and essential nutrients, such as vitamin B6 and potassium, which support digestion and overall health.
- Garlic, cumin, and chili powder contain anti-inflammatory properties and support immune function.

Preparation Time: 45 minutes

3: Lentil and Vegetable Soup

Ingredients:

- 1 cup dried green or brown lentils, rinsed
- 4 cups vegetable broth
- 1 onion, diced

- 2 carrots, diced

- 2 celery stalks, diced

- 2 cloves garlic, minced

- 1 teaspoon ground cumin

- 1/2 teaspoon ground turmeric

- 1/2 teaspoon paprika

- 1 bay leaf

- Salt and pepper to taste

- 2 tablespoons olive oil

- 2 tablespoons lemon juice

- Optional: chopped fresh parsley or cilantro for garnish

Instructions:

- In a large pot, heat olive oil over medium heat.

- Add diced onion, carrots, and celery to the pot. Sauté for 5-7 minutes until vegetables are softened.

- Add minced garlic, ground cumin, ground turmeric, paprika, and bay leaf to the pot. Cook for 1-2 minutes until fragrant.

- Add dried lentils and vegetable broth to the pot. Bring to a boil, then reduce heat to low, cover, and simmer for 20-25 minutes until lentils are tender.

- Once lentils are cooked, remove the bay leaf from the soup.

- Stir in lemon juice and season with salt and pepper to taste.

- Ladle the soup into serving bowls.

- If desired, garnish with chopped fresh parsley or cilantro.

- Serve hot and enjoy your hearty and nutritious lentil and vegetable soup!

Health Benefits:

- Lentils are rich in fiber, protein, and folate, which support digestion, blood sugar regulation, and liver health.

- Onions, carrots, celery, and garlic provide vitamins, minerals, and antioxidants that support immune function and liver detoxification.

- Spices like cumin, turmeric, and paprika have anti-inflammatory properties that support liver health and overall well-being.

- Olive oil provides healthy fats and antioxidants, which support heart health and inflammation.

- Lemon juice adds vitamin C and acidity, which enhance flavor and aid digestion.

Preparation Time: 30-35 minutes

4: Grilled Chicken with Quinoa and Steamed Broccoli

Ingredients:

- 2 boneless, skinless chicken breasts
- 1 cup quinoa, rinsed
- 2 cups water or chicken broth
- 2 cups broccoli florets
- 2 tablespoons olive oil
- 1 lemon, divided
- Salt and pepper to taste
- Optional: chopped fresh herbs (such as parsley or thyme) for garnish

Instructions:

- Preheat the grill to medium-high heat.

- Season the chicken breasts with salt, pepper, and a squeeze of lemon juice.

- Grill the chicken breasts for 6-8 minutes per side, or until cooked through and no longer pink in the center.

- While the chicken is grilling, in a saucepan, combine quinoa and water or chicken broth. Bring to a boil, then reduce heat to low, cover, and simmer for 15-20 minutes until quinoa is tender and water is absorbed.

- In a separate pot, steam broccoli florets until tender, about 5-7 minutes.

- Once the quinoa is cooked, fluff it with a fork and drizzle with olive oil and a squeeze of lemon juice. Season with salt and pepper to taste.

- Divide the cooked quinoa and steamed broccoli onto plates.

- Place grilled chicken breasts on top of the quinoa and broccoli.

- Garnish with chopped fresh herbs if desired.

- Serve hot and enjoy your flavorful grilled chicken with quinoa and steamed broccoli!

Health Benefits:

- Chicken breasts are a lean source of protein and provide essential amino acids that support muscle repair and overall health.
- Quinoa is a complete protein and contains fiber, vitamins, and minerals that support digestion and liver health.
- Broccoli is rich in antioxidants, fiber, and vitamins, such as vitamin C and vitamin K, which support immune function and liver detoxification.
- Olive oil provides healthy fats and antioxidants, which support heart health and inflammation.
- Lemon juice adds vitamin C and acidity, which enhance flavor and aid digestion.

Preparation Time: 30-35 minutes

5: Roasted Vegetable and Chickpea Buddha Bowl

Ingredients:

- 1 can (15 ounces) chickpeas, drained and rinsed

- 2 cups mixed vegetables (such as sweet potatoes, Brussels sprouts, cauliflower)

- 2 tablespoons olive oil

- 1 teaspoon garlic powder

- 1 teaspoon paprika

- Salt and pepper to taste

- 2 cups cooked quinoa or brown rice

- 1 avocado, sliced

- 2 tablespoons tahini

- Juice of 1 lemon

- Optional toppings: sesame seeds, chopped fresh parsley

Instructions:

- Preheat the oven to 400°F (200°C).

- Place chickpeas and mixed vegetables on a baking sheet lined with parchment paper.

- Drizzle olive oil over the chickpeas and vegetables, then sprinkle with garlic powder, paprika, salt, and pepper. Toss to coat evenly.

- Roast in the preheated oven for 25-30 minutes, stirring halfway through, until chickpeas are crispy and vegetables are tender.
- While the chickpeas and vegetables are roasting, prepare the quinoa or brown rice according to package instructions.
- In a small bowl, whisk together tahini and lemon juice to make the dressing.
- To assemble the Buddha bowls, divide cooked quinoa or brown rice among serving bowls.
- Top with roasted chickpeas and vegetables.
- Add sliced avocado on top.
- Drizzle with tahini dressing.
- Garnish with sesame seeds and chopped fresh parsley if desired.
- Serve warm and enjoy your nourishing roasted vegetable and chickpea Buddha bowl!

Health Benefits:

- Chickpeas are rich in protein, fiber, and essential nutrients, supporting digestion and liver health.

- Mixed vegetables provide vitamins, minerals, and antioxidants that support liver detoxification and overall well-being.

- Quinoa or brown rice offers fiber and complex carbohydrates for sustained energy and digestion.

- Avocado provides healthy fats and essential nutrients, such as potassium and vitamin E, which support heart health and inflammation.

- Tahini is rich in healthy fats, protein, and minerals, such as calcium and magnesium, which support bone health and liver function.

Preparation Time: 40 minutes

6: Turkey and Vegetable Stir-Fry

Ingredients:

- 1 lb (450g) turkey breast, thinly sliced

- 2 cups mixed vegetables (such as bell peppers, snap peas, carrots, mushrooms)

- 2 tablespoons olive oil

- 3 cloves garlic, minced

- 1 tablespoon grated fresh ginger

- 3 tablespoons low-sodium soy sauce or tamari

- 1 tablespoon rice vinegar

- 1 tablespoon honey or maple syrup

- 1 teaspoon sesame oil

- Cooked brown rice or quinoa for serving

- Optional toppings: sliced green onions, sesame seeds

Instructions:

- In a small bowl, whisk together soy sauce or tamari, rice vinegar, honey or maple syrup, and sesame oil to make the sauce. Set aside.

- Heat olive oil in a large skillet or wok over medium-high heat.

- Add sliced turkey breast to the skillet and cook for 3-4 minutes until browned.

- Remove the turkey from the skillet and set aside.

- In the same skillet, add minced garlic and grated ginger. Stir-fry for 1 minute until fragrant.

- Add mixed vegetables to the skillet and stir-fry for 5-7 minutes until crisp-tender.

- Return the cooked turkey to the skillet.

- Pour the sauce over the turkey and vegetables. Toss until everything is well coated and heated through.

- Serve the turkey and vegetable stir-fry over cooked brown rice or quinoa.
- Garnish with sliced green onions and sesame seeds if desired.
- Serve hot and enjoy your flavorful turkey and vegetable stir-fry!

Health Benefits:

- Turkey breast is a lean source of protein and contains essential amino acids that support muscle repair and overall health.
- Mixed vegetables provide vitamins, minerals, and antioxidants that support liver health and overall well-being.
- Garlic and ginger contain anti-inflammatory properties and support immune function.
- Soy sauce or tamari adds savory flavor while providing amino acids and minerals.
- Brown rice or quinoa offers fiber and complex carbohydrates for sustained energy and digestion.

Preparation Time: 30 minutes

7: Mediterranean Baked Cod with Roasted Vegetables

Ingredients:

- 2 cod fillets
- 2 cups mixed vegetables (such as zucchini, cherry tomatoes, red onion, bell peppers)
- 2 tablespoons olive oil
- 2 cloves garlic, minced
- 1 teaspoon dried oregano
- 1/2 teaspoon dried thyme
- Salt and pepper to taste
- Lemon wedges for serving
- Fresh parsley for garnish

Instructions:

- Preheat the oven to 400°F (200°C).
- Place cod fillets on a baking sheet lined with parchment paper.
- In a bowl, toss mixed vegetables with olive oil, minced garlic, dried oregano, dried thyme, salt, and pepper until evenly coated.

- Spread the vegetables around the cod fillets on the baking sheet.
- Bake in the preheated oven for 15-20 minutes, or until cod is cooked through and flakes easily with a fork.
- Remove from the oven and serve the baked cod with roasted vegetables.
- Squeeze fresh lemon juice over the cod before serving.
- Garnish with fresh parsley.
- Enjoy your flavorful and nutritious Mediterranean baked cod with roasted vegetables!

Health Benefits:

- Cod is a lean source of protein and provides essential nutrients, such as omega-3 fatty acids, which support heart health and reduce inflammation.
- Mixed vegetables provide a variety of vitamins, minerals, and antioxidants that support liver health and overall well-being.

- Olive oil offers heart-healthy monounsaturated fats and antioxidants, which support inflammation and liver health.

- Garlic, oregano, and thyme contain anti-inflammatory properties and support immune function.

Preparation Time: 25 minutes

8: Quinoa and Black Bean Stuffed Bell Peppers

Ingredients:

- 4 bell peppers, halved and seeds removed

- 1 cup cooked quinoa

- 1 can (15 ounces) black beans, drained and rinsed

- 1 cup corn kernels (fresh or frozen)

- 1 cup cherry tomatoes, halved

- 1/2 cup diced red onion

- 2 cloves garlic, minced

- 1 teaspoon ground cumin

- 1 teaspoon chili powder

- Salt and pepper to taste

- Optional toppings: sliced avocado, chopped fresh cilantro, Greek yogurt or sour cream

Instructions:

- Preheat the oven to 375°F (190°C).
- In a large bowl, combine cooked quinoa, black beans, corn kernels, cherry tomatoes, diced red onion, minced garlic, ground cumin, chili powder, salt, and pepper.
- Fill each halved bell pepper with the quinoa mixture.
- Place stuffed bell peppers in a baking dish.
- Cover the baking dish with foil and bake in the preheated oven for 25-30 minutes, or until bell peppers are tender.
- Remove from the oven and let cool slightly before serving.
- Serve the quinoa and black bean stuffed bell peppers with optional toppings such as sliced avocado, chopped fresh cilantro, and Greek yogurt or sour cream.
- Enjoy your flavorful and satisfying quinoa and black bean stuffed bell peppers!

Health Benefits:

- Quinoa provides protein, fiber, and essential nutrients, supporting digestion and liver health.
- Black beans offer protein, fiber, and antioxidants, supporting heart health and blood sugar regulation.
- Mixed vegetables provide vitamins, minerals, and antioxidants that support liver health and overall well-being.
- Garlic, cumin, and chili powder contain anti-inflammatory properties and support immune function.
- Avocado provides healthy fats and essential nutrients, such as potassium and vitamin E, which support heart health and inflammation.

Preparation Time: 40 minutes

9: Lemon Garlic Shrimp with Quinoa and Steamed Asparagus

Ingredients:

- 1 lb (450g) shrimp, peeled and deveined
- 2 cups cooked quinoa

- 1 lb (450g) asparagus, ends trimmed

- 2 tablespoons olive oil

- 4 cloves garlic, minced

- Zest and juice of 1 lemon

- Salt and pepper to taste

- Optional: chopped fresh parsley for garnish

Instructions:

- Preheat the oven to 400°F (200°C).

- Place the asparagus on a baking sheet and drizzle with 1 tablespoon of olive oil. Season with salt and pepper.

- Roast the asparagus in the preheated oven for 10-12 minutes, or until tender.

- While the asparagus is roasting, heat the remaining olive oil in a large skillet over medium heat.

- Add the minced garlic to the skillet and cook for 1-2 minutes until fragrant.

- Add the shrimp to the skillet and cook for 2-3 minutes on each side until pink and cooked through.

- Stir in the lemon zest and juice, and season with salt and pepper to taste.

- To serve, divide the cooked quinoa among plates, top with the lemon garlic shrimp, and serve with the roasted asparagus.
- Garnish with chopped fresh parsley if desired.
- Enjoy your delicious and light lemon garlic shrimp with quinoa and steamed asparagus!

Health Benefits:

- Shrimp is low in calories and fat, yet high in protein, making it a great option for weight management and muscle repair.
- Quinoa provides fiber, protein, and essential nutrients, supporting digestion and liver health.
- Asparagus is rich in antioxidants and vitamins, such as vitamin K and folate, which support liver detoxification and overall well-being.
- Olive oil contains heart-healthy monounsaturated fats and antioxidants, which support inflammation and liver health.
- Lemon adds vitamin C and acidity, enhancing flavor and aiding digestion.

Preparation Time: 25 minutes

Ingredients:

- 1 block (14-16 ounces) extra-firm tofu, cubed

- 2 cups mixed vegetables (such as bell peppers, broccoli, carrots, snap peas)

- 1 can (14 ounces) coconut milk

- 2 tablespoons red curry paste

- 2 tablespoons soy sauce or tamari

- 1 tablespoon coconut oil

- 2 cloves garlic, minced

- 1 tablespoon grated fresh ginger

- Juice of 1 lime

- Salt and pepper to taste

- Cooked brown rice for serving

- Optional toppings: chopped fresh cilantro, lime wedges

Instructions:

- Heat coconut oil in a large skillet or wok over medium heat.

- Add cubed tofu to the skillet and cook for 5-7 minutes, flipping occasionally, until golden brown and crispy on all sides. Remove tofu from the skillet and set aside.

- In the same skillet, add minced garlic and grated ginger. Cook for 1-2 minutes until fragrant.

- Add mixed vegetables to the skillet and stir-fry for 5-7 minutes until crisp-tender.

- Stir in red curry paste and cook for 1 minute, stirring constantly.

- Pour in coconut milk and soy sauce or tamari, stirring to combine.

- Add the cooked tofu back to the skillet and simmer for 5-7 minutes until vegetables are tender and tofu is heated through.

- Stir in lime juice, and season with salt and pepper to taste.

- Serve the tofu and vegetable coconut curry over cooked brown rice.

- Garnish with chopped fresh cilantro and lime wedges if desired.

- Enjoy your aromatic and flavorful tofu and vegetable coconut curry!

Health Benefits:

- Tofu provides plant-based protein and essential nutrients, supporting muscle repair and overall health.
- Mixed vegetables offer vitamins, minerals, and antioxidants that support liver health and overall well-being.
- Coconut milk contains healthy fats and medium-chain triglycerides, which support energy production and liver health.
- Garlic and ginger have anti-inflammatory properties and support immune function.
- Brown rice provides fiber and complex carbohydrates for sustained energy and digestion.

Preparation Time: 30 minutes

1: Avocado and Chickpea Mash on Whole Grain Crackers

Ingredients:

- 1 ripe avocado
- 1/2 cup cooked chickpeas, drained and rinsed
- 1 tablespoon lemon juice
- 1 clove garlic, minced
- Salt and pepper to taste
- Whole grain crackers for serving
- Optional toppings: sliced cherry tomatoes, chopped fresh parsley, red pepper flakes

Instructions:

- In a bowl, mash the ripe avocado with a fork until smooth.
- Add cooked chickpeas to the mashed avocado and mash them together until well combined.
- Stir in lemon juice, minced garlic, salt, and pepper to taste.

- Spread the avocado and chickpea mash onto whole grain crackers.
- If desired, top with sliced cherry tomatoes, chopped fresh parsley, or red pepper flakes for extra flavor.
- Serve immediately and enjoy your creamy and nutritious avocado and chickpea mash on whole grain crackers!

Health Benefits:

- Avocado is rich in healthy fats, vitamins, and minerals, such as vitamin E, potassium, and folate, which support heart health and liver function.
- Chickpeas provide protein, fiber, and essential nutrients, supporting digestion and blood sugar regulation.
- Whole grain crackers offer fiber and complex carbohydrates for sustained energy and digestion.
- Lemon juice adds vitamin C and acidity, enhancing flavor and aiding digestion.
- Garlic contains anti-inflammatory properties and supports immune function.

Preparation Time: 10 minutes

Ingredients:

- 1 cup Greek yogurt (plain or flavored)
- 1/2 cup mixed berries (such as strawberries, blueberries, raspberries)
- 2 tablespoons almonds, chopped
- 1 tablespoon honey or maple syrup (optional)
- Optional add-ins: chia seeds, granola, shredded coconut

Instructions:

- In a serving glass or bowl, layer Greek yogurt, mixed berries, and chopped almonds.
- If desired, drizzle honey or maple syrup over the layers for added sweetness.
- Repeat the layers until the glass or bowl is filled.
- Optionally, sprinkle chia seeds, granola, or shredded coconut on top for extra texture and flavor.

- Serve immediately and enjoy your refreshing and protein-packed Greek yogurt parfait with mixed berries and almonds!

Health Benefits:

- Greek yogurt is high in protein, probiotics, and calcium, which support digestive health and immune function.

- Mixed berries are rich in antioxidants, vitamins, and fiber, which support heart health and liver detoxification.

- Almonds provide healthy fats, protein, and essential nutrients, such as vitamin E and magnesium, which support brain health and inflammation.

- Honey or maple syrup (if added) offer natural sweetness and antioxidants, enhancing flavor without added refined sugars.

- Optional add-ins like chia seeds, granola, or shredded coconut add fiber, texture, and additional nutrients to the parfait.

Preparation Time: 5 minutes

3: Cucumber and Hummus Stacks

Ingredients:

- 1 large cucumber
- 1/2 cup hummus (store-bought or homemade)
- Cherry tomatoes, sliced (for garnish)
- Fresh basil leaves (for garnish)
- Balsamic glaze (optional, for drizzling)

Instructions:

- Wash the cucumber and cut it into thin rounds.
- Take a cucumber round and spread a thin layer of hummus on top.
- Place another cucumber round on top of the hummus to create a stack.
- Continue layering cucumber rounds and hummus until you have a stack of desired height.
- Garnish the top of each stack with a slice of cherry tomato and a fresh basil leaf.
- If desired, drizzle balsamic glaze over the stacks for added flavor.
- Repeat the process to make more cucumber and hummus stacks.

- Serve immediately and enjoy your refreshing and crunchy snack!

Health Benefits:

- Cucumber is hydrating and low in calories, while also providing vitamins and minerals that support hydration and liver function.
- Hummus is a good source of plant-based protein and fiber, which helps keep you feeling full and supports digestion.
- Cherry tomatoes are rich in antioxidants and vitamins, particularly vitamin C, which supports immune function and liver detoxification.
- Basil leaves add flavor and also provide antioxidants and anti-inflammatory compounds that support overall health.

Preparation Time: 10 minutes

4: Almond Butter and Banana Rice Cakes

Ingredients:

- Rice cakes (plain or whole grain)
- Almond butter (or any nut or seed butter of choice)

- 1 ripe banana, sliced

- Honey (optional, for drizzling)

- Cinnamon (optional, for sprinkling)

Instructions:

- Spread a generous amount of almond butter on each rice cake.

- Top the almond butter with slices of ripe banana.

- Drizzle honey over the banana slices, if desired, for added sweetness.

- Sprinkle a pinch of cinnamon over the top for extra flavor, if desired.

- Repeat the process to make more almond butter and banana rice cakes.

- Serve immediately and enjoy your delicious and satisfying snack!

Health Benefits:

- Rice cakes provide a light and crunchy base for the snack, while also being low in calories and gluten-free.

- Almond butter is rich in healthy fats, protein, and fiber, which help keep you feeling full and satisfied between meals.

- Banana slices add natural sweetness and provide vitamins, minerals, and fiber that support digestion and liver health.

- Honey (if added) offers natural sweetness and antioxidants, while cinnamon adds flavor and may help regulate blood sugar levels.

Preparation Time: 5 minutes

5: Kale Chips

Ingredients:

- 1 bunch of kale
- 1 tablespoon olive oil
- Salt to taste
- Optional seasonings: garlic powder, onion powder, paprika, nutritional yeast

Instructions:

- Preheat the oven to 275°F (135°C).

- Wash and thoroughly dry the kale leaves. Remove the stems and tear the leaves into bite-sized pieces.
- In a large bowl, toss the kale leaves with olive oil until evenly coated.
- Spread the kale leaves in a single layer on a baking sheet lined with parchment paper.
- Sprinkle salt and any desired seasonings over the kale leaves.
- Bake in the preheated oven for 20-25 minutes, or until the kale is crispy and edges are lightly browned.
- Remove from the oven and let cool slightly before serving.
- Enjoy your homemade kale chips as a crunchy and nutritious snack!

Health Benefits:

- Kale is a nutrient-dense leafy green vegetable rich in vitamins A, C, and K, as well as antioxidants and fiber, which support liver health and detoxification.
- Olive oil provides healthy fats and antioxidants, which support heart health and inflammation.

- Seasonings like garlic powder, onion powder, paprika, and nutritional yeast add flavor without extra calories or unhealthy ingredients.

Preparation Time: 30 minutes

6: Chia Pudding with Mixed Berries

Ingredients:

- 2 tablespoons chia seeds
- 1/2 cup unsweetened almond milk (or any milk of choice)
- 1/2 teaspoon vanilla extract
- 1 teaspoon honey or maple syrup (optional)
- 1/2 cup mixed berries (such as strawberries, blueberries, raspberries)

Instructions:

- In a small bowl or jar, mix together chia seeds, almond milk, vanilla extract, and honey or maple syrup if using.
- Stir well to combine, ensuring there are no clumps of chia seeds.

- Cover the bowl or jar and refrigerate for at least 2 hours, or preferably overnight, to allow the chia seeds to thicken and absorb the liquid.
- Once the chia pudding has set, give it a stir to redistribute the chia seeds.
- Spoon the chia pudding into serving bowls or jars.
- Top with mixed berries.
- Serve chilled and enjoy your creamy and nutritious chia pudding with mixed berries!

Health Benefits:

- Chia seeds are rich in fiber, omega-3 fatty acids, and antioxidants, which support digestion, heart health, and liver function.
- Almond milk is low in calories and provides vitamins and minerals, such as vitamin E and calcium, which support bone health and liver function.
- Vanilla extract adds flavor without extra calories or unhealthy ingredients.
- Mixed berries are rich in antioxidants, vitamins, and fiber, which support immune function and liver detoxification.

- Honey or maple syrup (if added) offer natural sweetness and antioxidants, enhancing flavor without added refined sugars.

Preparation Time: 5 minutes (plus chilling time)

7: Roasted Chickpeas

Ingredients:

- 1 can (15 ounces) chickpeas (garbanzo beans), drained and rinsed
- 1 tablespoon olive oil
- 1 teaspoon ground cumin
- 1 teaspoon smoked paprika
- 1/2 teaspoon garlic powder
- Salt to taste

Instructions:

- Preheat the oven to 400°F (200°C).
- Rinse and drain the chickpeas, then pat them dry with a clean towel or paper towels.
- In a bowl, toss the chickpeas with olive oil until evenly coated.

- Add ground cumin, smoked paprika, garlic powder, and salt to the chickpeas. Toss until the chickpeas are coated with the spices.

- Spread the seasoned chickpeas in a single layer on a baking sheet lined with parchment paper.

- Roast in the preheated oven for 25-30 minutes, or until the chickpeas are golden brown and crispy.

- Remove from the oven and let cool slightly before serving.

- Enjoy your crunchy and flavorful roasted chickpeas as a healthy snack!

Health Benefits:

- Chickpeas are rich in fiber, protein, and essential nutrients, supporting digestion and blood sugar regulation.

- Olive oil provides healthy fats and antioxidants, which support heart health and inflammation.

- Ground cumin, smoked paprika, and garlic powder add flavor without extra calories or unhealthy ingredients.

Preparation Time: 35-40 minutes

8: Apple Slices with Almond Butter and Cinnamon

Ingredients:

- 1 apple, cored and sliced
- 2 tablespoons almond butter (or any nut or seed butter of choice)
- Ground cinnamon for sprinkling

Instructions:

- Core the apple and slice it into thin rounds or wedges.
- Spread almond butter on each apple slice.
- Sprinkle ground cinnamon over the almond butter.
- Repeat the process for each apple slice.
- Arrange the apple slices on a plate or serving dish.
- Serve immediately and enjoy your crunchy, creamy, and naturally sweet apple slices with almond butter and cinnamon!

Health Benefits:

- Apples are a good source of fiber, vitamins, and antioxidants, which support digestion and heart health.

- Almond butter provides healthy fats, protein, and essential nutrients, helping to keep you feeling full and satisfied.
- Cinnamon adds flavor and may help regulate blood sugar levels.

Preparation Time: 5 minutes

9: Carrot and Hummus Dip

Ingredients:

- 2 large carrots, peeled and sliced into sticks
- 1/2 cup hummus (store-bought or homemade)
- Fresh parsley or cilantro for garnish (optional)

Instructions:

- Wash, peel, and slice the carrots into sticks.
- Arrange the carrot sticks on a serving plate.
- Place the hummus in a small bowl in the center of the plate.
- Garnish the hummus with fresh parsley or cilantro if desired.

- Serve immediately and enjoy dipping the carrot sticks into the hummus for a crunchy and nutritious snack!

Health Benefits:

- Carrots are rich in beta-carotene, vitamins, and antioxidants that support liver health and overall well-being.
- Hummus provides plant-based protein, fiber, and healthy fats, which help keep you feeling full and satisfied between meals.
- Fresh herbs like parsley or cilantro add flavor and may have detoxifying properties that support liver function.

Preparation Time: 5 minutes

10: Seaweed Snack Rolls with Avocado

Ingredients:

- 2 sheets of nori seaweed
- 1 ripe avocado, thinly sliced
- Sesame seeds for garnish (optional)

Instructions:

- Lay out a sheet of nori seaweed on a clean surface.
- Place thinly sliced avocado along one edge of the nori sheet.
- Roll up the nori sheet tightly, enclosing the avocado slices.
- Repeat the process with the second sheet of nori and remaining avocado slices.
- Use a sharp knife to slice each roll into bite-sized pieces.
- Sprinkle sesame seeds over the seaweed rolls for garnish if desired.
- Serve immediately and enjoy your crunchy and savory seaweed snack rolls with avocado!

Health Benefits:

- Nori seaweed is low in calories and rich in vitamins, minerals, and antioxidants, including iodine, which supports thyroid function and liver health.
- Avocado provides healthy fats, vitamins, and minerals, such as potassium and vitamin E, which support heart health and inflammation.

Preparation Time: 10 minutes

CONCLUSION

Liver cleanse diet recipes provide a valuable approach for women seeking to enhance their liver health and overall vitality.

These recipes are specifically crafted to include ingredients rich in antioxidants, vitamins, and minerals that are essential for detoxifying and supporting liver function.

Integrating these meals into your daily diet can lead to noticeable improvements in energy, clearer skin, and better digestion, contributing to a greater sense of well-being.

By focusing on whole, unprocessed foods, these liver cleanse recipes help reduce the burden on the liver, allowing it to repair and rejuvenate more effectively.

Whether you're looking to reset your dietary habits, manage weight, or simply give your body a healthful boost, these recipes can be a cornerstone in your pursuit of a healthier lifestyle.

Encouraging regular incorporation of these cleansing meals can create lasting habits that not only improve liver health but also enhance your overall health profile.

As you embark on this journey, be mindful of your body's responses and enjoy the varied, delicious options that support liver health.

Embrace this path as a proactive step towards a more energized and vibrant life.

www.ingramcontent.com/pod-product-compliance
Lightning Source LLC
Chambersburg PA
CBHW050811250726

48653CB00006B/2171